COMPLETE GUIDE TO METHYLENE BLUE

The Methylene Blue Breakthrough: Exploring The Therapeutic Potential Of Methylene Blue & Navigating Its Scientific And Medical Frontiers

DOMINIC ROBERT

Table of Contents

Introductory

There are several applications for the synthetic dye and medicine known as methylene blue. The following is a list of its most important interpretations:

• Stain for Biological Tissues and Cells: Methylene Blue is a well-known biological stain that is frequently utilized in laboratories for the purpose of staining biological tissues and cells. It is possible to use it in microbiology, as well as in histology and cytology, in order to improve the visibility of particular structures when viewed via a microscope.

• Medication: Methylene Blue is used in the medical field for a variety of therapeutic uses. Methemoglobinemia, a disorder in which the amount of oxygen that hemoglobin is capable of carrying in its molecules, can be treated using this substance. Methylene Blue is a reducing chemical that plays a role in the process of converting methemoglobin back into normal hemoglobin.

• Methylene Blue has antibacterial properties, and it may be utilized in that capacity in certain contexts. It has been administered topically to wounds, and it is considered to contain qualities that inhibit the growth of microbes.

• Methylene Blue is also utilized as a diagnostic agent within the context of the medical field. It can be utilized in a variety of diagnostic processes and tests to assist in the identification of specific conditions.

• Antimalarial Agent: Currently, studies are being conducted to investigate the viability of using methylene blue as an antimalarial agent. It has been demonstrated to be effective in preventing the growth of the parasites that cause malaria.

Methylene Blue does have therapeutic applications; however, due to the possibility of adverse effects and combinations with other medications, it should only be used under the supervision of a qualified medical practitioner. It is vital to keep in mind this fact.

CHAPTER ONE

Methylene Blue's Chemical Composition

Methylene Blue has a complicated chemical structure, and its systematic name is 3,7-bis(dimethylamino)phenothiazin-5-ium chloride. This name comes from the chemical formula. Let's have a look at the fundamental building blocks of its chemical structure:

• Phenothiazine Ring System Methylene Blue's structure is built around a phenothiazine ring system in its center. This structure is made up of three rings of benzene bonded together with a five-membered ring containing sulfur.

• Dimethylamino Groups: The phenothiazine ring system has two dimethylamino (N(CH3)2) groups linked to it. These groups are referred to as the dimethylamino groups. The functional groups nitrogen and methyl (CH3) can be found in these groupings.

• Group Comprised of Quaternary Ammonium Ions The nitrogen atoms that are found in the dimethylamino groups are quaternary ammonium ions, which means that they have a positive charge.

• Chloride Ion: Methylene Blue is most commonly found in the form of a chloride salt. In this form, a chloride ion, denoted by the symbol Cl-, is coupled with the positively charged quaternary ammonium groups. The overall charge of the molecule is helped to be more stable by the presence of the chloride ion.

It is common practice to write the chemical formula for methylene blue as $C16H18ClN3S$. This formula indicates the number of atoms in the molecule as well as their kinds.

The substance in question is a cationic dye, which indicates that it possesses a positive charge. Because it both absorbs and reflects particular wavelengths of light, methylene blue has a blue color because of this combination of properties.

Because of its capacity to both receive and contribute electrons, methylene blue is useful in a wide variety of applications. These uses include coloring biological samples, treating medical diseases, and acting as a redox indicator in chemical reactions. Methylene blue's versatility is owing to its ability to absorb and donate electrons.

Various Applications In Medicine

Because of its qualities as a dye, redox agent, and possible therapeutic agent, methylene blue has a variety of applications in the medical field. The following are some of its key applications in medicine:

• Methemoglobinemia treatment: Methemoglobinemia is a disorder in which the oxygen-carrying molecule in red blood cells, hemoglobin, is unable to release oxygen in an efficient manner. This results in methemoglobinemia. Methylene Blue is a reducing chemical that can convert methemoglobin back into normal hemoglobin, which will then restore the oxygen-carrying capability of the blood. In times of crisis, intravenous administration is frequently the method of choice.

• Diagnostic Tool Methylene Blue is a substance that has the potential to be utilized in a variety of medical operations as a diagnostic tool. During histological exams, it is utilized to detect and stain specific features in the tissues or cells that are being examined. For instance, it can be put to use to bring attention to the nucleus of cells when viewed under a microscope.

• Antidote for Cyanide Poisoning Methylene Blue has the potential to be utilized as an antidote in some situations involving cyanide poisoning. It accomplishes this by facilitating the transformation of cyanide into compounds with lower toxicity.

• Photodynamic Therapy (PDT): The use of methylene blue as a component of photodynamic therapy, a potential treatment for some forms of cancer, has been the subject of research. In this application, the production of reactive oxygen species, which can harm and kill cancer cells, is triggered by the exposure of Methylene Blue to light.

- Antimalarial Research: Currently, there is research being conducted that is looking into the possibility of using methylene blue as an antimalarial agent. It has demonstrated some degree of success in reducing the growth of the parasite that causes malaria, known as Plasmodium.

Methylene Blue does have therapeutic applications; nevertheless, its usage should be carefully monitored and administered by healthcare experts due to the possibility for adverse effects and interactions.

It is crucial to note this, as it is vital to note that while Methylene Blue does have therapeutic applications. The individual medical problem that is being treated determines the appropriate dosage and administration.

Utilized In The Fields Of Medicine And Surgery

In the fields of medicine and surgery, methylene blue can be used in a variety of contexts. The following are some of its applications:

• Treatment for Methemoglobinemia

Methylene Blue is used as a treatment for methemoglobinemia, a condition in which the blood contains a high quantity of methemoglobin, which is unable to transfer oxygen in an efficient manner. The oxygen-carrying capacity of the blood is restored when methemoglobin is converted back to normal hemoglobin by the reducing power of methylene blue.

• Visualization of the Anatomy Methylene Blue is a substance that may be utilized during surgical procedures for the purpose of visualizing various anatomical components. During operations, for instance, it may be injected into lymph nodes or vessels in order to provide assistance to surgeons in identifying and mapping the lymphatic system or blood vessels.

• In cancer surgery, notably for breast cancer and melanoma, methylene blue is occasionally used to detect sentinel lymph nodes. This is done through a process known as sentinel lymph node mapping. A primary tumor's cancer cells are most likely to spread to these lymph nodes initially after they have disseminated to other lymph nodes. By injecting methylene blue close to the tumor, surgeons are able to locate sentinel lymph nodes and remove them for further investigation.

• During thyroid and parathyroid procedures, the dye methylene blue can be used as a tool to assist in the identification of the patient's parathyroid glands. This helps to prevent the inadvertent removal of these vital glands, which are responsible for regulating calcium levels throughout the body.

• Methylene Blue is able to detect and visualize some fistulas, which are aberrant connections between organs or tissues. This is accomplished by its use in fistula detection. It can either be injected or given topically in order to assist surgeons in identifying the presence of fistulas as well as their location.

• Visualization of the Ureters Methylene Blue is a substance that can be utilized in urological treatments in order to identify and image the ureters. Having this information on hand is especially useful for surgery involving the urinary bladder or the reproductive organs.

• Methylene Blue Is Used to Treat Vasoplegic Syndrome Methylene Blue has been used in cardiac surgery to treat vasoplegic syndrome, a disorder that is characterized by very low blood pressure despite normal or high cardiac output. In circumstances like these, it has the potential to assist in improving vascular tone and blood pressure.

It is essential to emphasize that the use of methylene blue in medicine and surgery should be carefully considered and delivered by professionals in the medical field. In addition, the potential benefits of using methylene blue should be weighed against the potential adverse effects and contraindications of using the substance.

CHAPTER TWO
Biological Repercussions

Because of the chemical qualities it possesses, methylene blue has a number of consequences on living organisms. Several of these consequences include the following:

• Methylene Blue is a redox-active molecule, which means it is capable of both accepting and donating electrons. This characteristic of the compound gives it its name. In the treatment of disorders such as methemoglobinemia, where it serves as a reducing agent to convert methemoglobin back to normal hemoglobin, this feature is employed.

• Antioxidant qualities: Methylene Blue has the ability to scavenge free radicals and possesses antioxidant qualities. Because of this, it has the potential to be useful in conditions that include high levels of oxidative stress.

• Methylene Blue's ability to inhibit nitric oxide synthase, an enzyme that plays a role in the creation of nitric oxide, is one of the compound's most important properties. This feature is relevant in cases when excessive nitric oxide generation contributes to pathophysiology. One example of such a disease is the vasoplegic syndrome, which can occur following cardiac surgery.

• Photodynamic Activity: When it is illuminated by light, methylene blue is capable of displaying photodynamic activity. It is utilized in the field of photodynamic therapy, where it is triggered by light to produce reactive oxygen species, which when directed at certain cells, such as cancer cells, can cause damage and death to those cells.

• Staining of Biological Structures: Methylene Blue is a chemical that is frequently used in research facilities as a biological stain. Its purpose is to improve the visibility of specific structures found within cells and tissues. Staining components such as nuclei can be done with it, which is helpful for microscopy and histology tests.

• Activity Against Certain Bacteria and Parasites Methylene Blue has been shown to possess some antibacterial activity against certain bacteria and parasites. Research has been conducted into the possibility that it could be used as a treatment for diseases such as malaria.

• Neuroprotective properties: Studies on the neuroprotective properties of methylene blue are still being conducted. It has been investigated for the possibility of slowing the progression of neurodegenerative disorders and the cognitive loss that comes with advancing age.

It is essential to highlight that although methylene blue has the potential to be used as a therapeutic agent, its application should be carefully controlled and monitored, especially when it comes to medical uses.

The patient being treated must be evaluated first before any decisions can be made regarding dosage or route of administration. Additionally, Methylene Blue, like any other chemical, has the potential to have adverse consequences; therefore, its use should only be undertaken under the guidance of trained medical specialists.

Diagnostic Applications

There are several diagnostic applications for methylene blue in a variety of sectors. The following is a list of some of its applications:

• Staining in Microbiology and Histology: Methylene Blue is a stain that is frequently used in both microbiology and histology. In order to improve the visibility of particular structures under a microscope, it can be applied to biological materials such as cells and tissues. In the field of microbiology, it is frequently utilized as a stain for the purpose of identifying microorganisms.

• Methylene Blue is a stain that can be used in cytology's nuclear staining procedure. This procedure makes cell nuclei more apparent when seen via a microscope. This is especially helpful in cytology research, which must necessarily include an investigation of the appearance and organization of individual cells.

- Staining and Identifying Nerve Fibers: Methylene Blue is a chemical that has been used in the field of neurology to stain and identify nerve fibers. It is possible to apply it to neural tissues, which makes the investigation of neuronal connections and structures much simpler.

- The Ziehl-Neelsen stain method is used for the detection of acid-fast bacteria, including Mycobacterium species, which are responsible for illnesses such as tuberculosis. Methylene Blue is used in this approach. Detection of Acid-fast Bacteria Methylene Blue is used in this method. The practice of clinical microbiology makes extensive use of this staining method.

• Ophthalmic Use of Methylene Blue for Vital Staining of the Cornea Methylene Blue is used in ophthalmology for vital staining of the cornea. It may be easier to see any imperfections or irregularities on the corneal surface as a result.

• In surgical operations, particularly those involving oncology, methylene blue can be injected close to a tumor in order to map the lymphatic drainage. This is done in order to locate lymph nodes. This helps identify and locate sentinel lymph nodes, which is helpful for both the stage of cancer and the planning of surgical procedures.

• Methylene Blue is a staining agent that can be utilized in surgical procedures involving the thyroid and the parathyroid glands in order to detect and differentiate parathyroid glands from the surrounding tissues. This helps to ensure that these vital glands are not accidentally removed from the patient during surgery.

• Methylene Blue is a useful tool for locating fistulas, which are aberrant connections between organs or tissues. Fistulas can be detected with this dye. The dye can be injected, and the surgeons will be able to identify the presence of the fistula as well as its precise position thanks to the appearance of the dye at a predetermined spot.

It is essential to keep in mind that the precise diagnostic use of methylene blue shifts depending on the circumstances as well as the kind of test or operation that is being carried out. The dye's capacity to stain and improve visibility makes it an extremely useful tool in a variety of medical and scientific contexts.

CHAPTER THREE
Utilizations In Medicine

Methylene Blue is utilized for a variety of therapeutic purposes across a wide range of medical specialties. Listed below are some of its most important applications in therapeutics:

• Treatment for Methemoglobinemia Methylene Blue is an essential component of the treatment for methemoglobinemia, a disorder in which hemoglobin is unable to transfer oxygen to tissues in an efficient manner. The oxygen-carrying ability of methemoglobin is restored when it is exposed to methylene blue, which functions as a reducing agent. This results in methemoglobin being converted back to normal hemoglobin (Fe2+).

• Antidote for Cyanide Poisoning The antidote for cyanide poisoning is known as methylene blue, and it can be utilized in some instances. It does this by encouraging the transformation of cyanide into compounds with a lower toxicity level, which helps to mitigate the negative effects of cyanide poisoning.

• Vasoplegic Syndrome During Cardiac Surgery Methylene Blue is used during cardiac surgery to treat vasoplegic syndrome, which is a condition characterized by severe hypotension despite normal or high cardiac output. Methylene Blue is used to treat vasoplegic syndrome. In these kinds of situations, Methylene Blue can be helpful in raising blood pressure by blocking nitric oxide synthase and increasing the tone of the blood vessels.

• Photodynamic Therapy for Cancer: Research is being done on the possibility of using methylene blue in photodynamic therapy, also known as PDT, for treating certain forms of cancer. Methylene Blue creates reactive oxygen species after being triggered by light; these species are capable of damaging and destroying cancer cells that are specifically targeted.

• Antimalarial Agent: Research has investigated the use of methylene blue to determine its potential as an antimalarial agent. It has showed some promise in preventing the growth of the parasites that cause malaria, and its potential use in combination treatments for the disease is currently the subject of research.

• Neuroprotective properties: Studies on the neuroprotective properties of methylene blue are still being conducted. It has been investigated for the possibility that it could slow or stop the progression of neurodegenerative disorders such as Alzheimer's and Parkinson's.

• Methylene Blue possesses antioxidant qualities, which allow it to neutralize potentially harmful free radicals in the body. This feature is useful in circumstances where oxidative stress plays a role, such as in certain neurodegenerative disorders, and it is advantageous in general.

It is essential to emphasize that although methylene blue has the potential to be used as a therapeutic agent, its application should be carefully regulated and monitored by trained medical personnel. It is necessary to take into account the particular medical condition that is being treated when making decisions regarding dosage, administration, and potential adverse effects.

The Risks Involved And Their Effects

When used properly and in accordance with the directions provided by qualified medical practitioners, methylene blue is generally regarded as safe. On the other hand, much like any other chemical or medication, it has the potential for both beneficial and adverse consequences. The following are some things to keep in mind with relation to the safety of methylene blue and its potential adverse effects:

Common adverse effects include:

• Urine That Turns Blue or Green Methylene Blue can cause a discoloration of the urine, which can take on a blue or green hue. This is one of the most obvious negative effects of the drug. This is an expected and very safe side effect.

Less Frequent Adverse Reactions:

• Nausea and Vomiting: After receiving Methylene Blue, some

people may have feelings of nausea or vomiting.

• Headache and dizziness are two potential adverse effects that, while not very common, are nonetheless a possibility.

• Pain at the Injection Site If methylene blue is given via injection, there is a chance that the patient will experience pain or discomfort at the injection site.

Rare but Potentially Serious Adverse Effects:

• When Methylene Blue is used in conjunction with other treatments that can alter serotonin levels, there is a possibility of developing a disease known as serotonin syndrome, which can be a potentially life-threatening condition. When Methylene Blue is used as a therapy for methemoglobinemia in combination with serotonergic medications, the chance of this side effect is significantly increased.

• Allergic Reactions: Although they are uncommon, Methylene Blue has been known to provoke allergic reactions in certain people. Rash, itching, swelling, severe disorientation, or difficulty breathing are some of the symptoms that could occur.

• Hemolysis: Methylene Blue has the potential to cause hemolysis in individuals who are deficient in glucose-6-phosphate dehydrogenase (G6PD). Hemolysis is the disintegration of red blood cells, which ultimately results in anemia. In certain populations, a G6PD deficiency is more prevalent than in others.

A Few Words About Safety and Priorities:

• Because it can raise the risk of serotonin syndrome, methylene blue should be used with extreme caution in patients who are also on serotonergic medicines (for example, certain antidepressants).

• As was indicated earlier, individuals who have a glucose-6-phosphate dehydrogenase (G6PD) deficit should exercise extreme caution when using this medication.

• Because the safety of its use during pregnancy and lactation has not been well researched, individuals who are pregnant or nursing should discuss the use of methylene blue with their primary care physician before beginning treatment.

• Because of the potential for interactions between Methylene Blue and other drugs, it is imperative that patients inform their healthcare providers about all medications and supplements they are currently taking.

• The dosage and route of administration of methylene blue should be set by qualified medical specialists with reference to the ailment that is being treated.

It is extremely important for individuals to contact their healthcare professional as soon as possible if they experience any unusual or severe side effects. This material is not exhaustive; precise warnings and concerns may vary depending on the individual's existing health issues as well as the situation in which they will be using methylene blue. Always seek the counsel and direction of a qualified healthcare practitioner for the most tailored care.

CHAPTER FOUR

Instructions For Use, Including Dosage And Administration

The dosage and administration of methylene blue is something that should be determined by a qualified medical expert, as it is dependent on the particular medical problem that is being treated. The following is a list of some general recommendations and things to keep in mind when using methylene blue:

The Treatment for Methemoglobinemia Is:

• Administration Via the Intravenous Route In order to treat methemoglobinemia, methylene blue is commonly given to the patient via the intravenous route (IV).

• The severity of the methemoglobinemia and the patient's weight are taken into consideration while determining the appropriate dosage. In most cases, it is administered with a gradual injection.

Poisoning from Cyanide:

• Administration Via Intravenous Route Methylene Blue, which is used as an antidote for cyanide poisoning, is given to the patient via intravenous route.

• Dosage: A healthcare expert will calculate the appropriate dosage for you based on the degree of poisoning you are experiencing.

Syndrome of Vasoplegia During Cardiac Surgery :

• Intravenous Administration In order to treat vasoplegic syndrome, the medication methylene blue is given to the patient intravenously during cardiac surgery.

• Dosage: The patient's condition and reaction to therapy are taken into consideration when determining the appropriate dosage.

Cancer Treatment Using Photodynamic Therapy:

- Administration Via the Skin or Intravenously Depending on the Cancer Treatment Protocol, Methylene Blue may be administered either via the skin (via topical application) or the veins (via intravenous injection) before to exposure to light.

- Dosage Both the amount of medication taken and how it is given are determined by the type and stage of cancer that is being treated.

Research on Malaria Treatment:

• Administration Via Mouth or Intravenous Route In the context of studies investigating the efficacy of methylene blue as an antimalarial drug, the substance may be given either orally or intravenously.

• Dosage: Dosages might vary widely depending on the research methodology and the particular study that is being conducted.

Regarding the correct dosage and route of administration of methylene blue, it is essential to adhere to the instructions provided by trained medical specialists. Self-administration or deviating from the doses that were given can result in undesirable side effects.

Watching and Taking Safety Measures:

• During the delivery of methylene blue, patients will be under the strict observation of medical professionals, who will be looking for any unpleasant responses or side effects.

• When combined with serotonergic drugs, the use of methylene blue should be approached with extreme caution due to the possibility of causing serotonin syndrome.

Before receiving Methylene Blue treatment, patients are encouraged to discuss with their healthcare professionals any pre-existing medical issues, medications they are currently taking, or potential allergies they may have. In addition, those who are getting Methylene Blue should be aware of its potential side effects and bad reactions, and they should report them as soon as possible.

Summary

Methylene Blue is a chemical that has many uses in the medical field, including diagnostics, surgery, and medicine more generally. Because of its redox qualities, it is useful in the treatment of methemoglobinemia and cyanide poisoning.

Additionally, because of its staining powers, it is utilized in histology, microbiology, and surgical operations. Methylene Blue may have potential medical applications for the treatment of a variety of illnesses, including vasoplegic syndrome, some tumors treated with photodynamic therapy, and current research into applications for neuroprotection and antimalarial treatment.

The use of Methylene Blue under the supervision of trained medical personnel is widely accepted to be risk-free; yet, it is not without the potential for adverse effects.

Urine turning a darker shade is one of the most typical adverse effects; other side effects, such as nausea and vomiting, may also occur. Even if they are uncommon, serious adverse effects including serotonin syndrome and allergic reactions still need to be taken into consideration.

Both the dosage and the manner in which methylene blue is administered change depending on the ailment that is being treated; therefore, it is essential that medical practitioners carefully monitor their patients.

Patients need to make sure that their healthcare providers are aware of any pre-existing diseases, drugs, or concerns that they have. This will ensure that treatment is both safe and successful.

The relevance of methylene blue in the field of medicine is highlighted by the fact that it possesses a wide variety of uses, ranging from that of a diagnostic stain to that of a therapeutic agent. Our current understanding of this molecule and its potential contributions to healthcare could be further expanded if further study reveals additional applications and advantages of the compound.

THE END